SWITCHBOARD SHIFT

SWITCHBOARD SHIFT

Poems

Kathleen Fagley

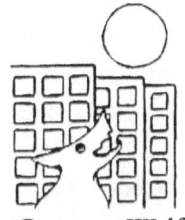

Concrete Wolf
Chapbook Award Series

Copyright © 2024 Kathleen Fagley

All rights reserved. No part of this publication may be reproduced, distributed, or transmitted in any form or by any means whatsoever without written permission from the publisher, except in the case of brief excerpts for critical reviews and articles. All inquiries should be addressed to Concrete Wolf Press.

Concrete Wolf Chapbook Award Series

Poetry
ISBN 978-1-936657-92-6

Cover art: Oklahoma Historical Society, Women Operating a Switchboard
OHS Photo Catalog: okhistory.org/research/collections/photos.html

Author photo by Tim Wessel

Design: Tonya Namura using American Typewriter and Adobe Garamond Pro

Concrete Wolf
PO Box 2220
Newport, OR 97365-0163

http://ConcreteWolf.com

ConcreteWolfPress@gmail.com

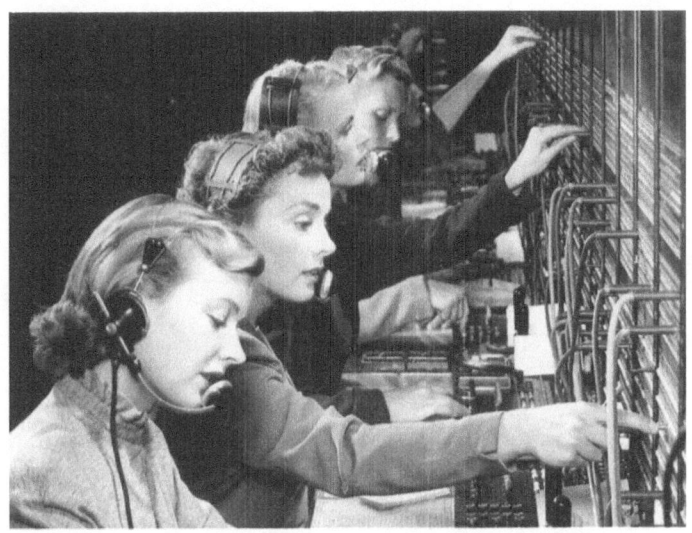

This book is dedicated to all the switchboard operators who keep the lines of communication open day and night in hospitals. Through storms and floods, crises, trauma, codes, the switchboard operator is the voice that can help you or your loved ones.

Contents

Getting Ready	1
Text Fields	3
Untethered	4
All Fall to Earth	5
First Disaster	6
First Code	7
Security	8
The Hospital as Halfway House	9
Code Red	10
Panic Buttons	11
Calling Codes	12
Lifeline™ Calls	14
Weekend Call Sheets	16
The Vigil	17
Overheard	18
Crash	19
How Did You Do That?	20
Voices	21
Hearing Test	22
Harvesting	23
After-Life	24
STAT	25
Self-Revelation	27
Loud the Silence	28
For Liesbet	29
After the After-Hours Clinic Closes	30
Misreads (at the Switchboard)	32
Late Shift	33
Acknowledgments	35
About the Author	37

SWITCHBOARD SHIFT

Getting Ready

Atomic and Greenwich Mean Time
do not reconcile on my board.
Am I seven minutes late or four?
I choose Greenwich Mean Time.
I have straddled that line.
Memories of the observatory,
and Queen's hunting ground puts me
in an English frame of mind
before the "Hello"
voice reaches me.

I position the mouthpiece, earpieces,
the metal band slips on silky hair.
My problem is that I have this pain,
behind my right testicle and I only have one.
I suggest Fast Track as an option
faster and less expensive if
he feels it is an emergency.
I add a caveat—there is always
a caveat—
You will need to be triaged of course,
that word again, *triaged*: French
for separating out. I think of culling
tiny stones from lentils.

If we follow our script,
if the astronomic signs are propitious,
I will have time to answer questions
and pronounce each word clearly,
supplying the missing parts of the sentences
reading the ellipsis, dash, punctuation marks
into the voices before they cut me off
or before I escape with one keystroke,

sending them away to another extension,
most likely an automated voice.

Slow down and take a deep breath, I tell myself,
there are twelve lines stacking up in the queue.
I use my first name but never
to the doctor who always asks
for me to stay on the line until
he reaches a real human being.

Text Fields

Board lights up, then digits flash
before I hear the voices:
a man with stomach pains,
a woman blew out her knee,
another I have to tell to speak up,
her baby hasn't moved for 24 hours.
She is seven and half months pregnant.

Eight hours of this and I feel as if
my ears are stopped up with water,
I feel the pain of these voices.

The doctor leans against the wall
between two rooms, the alpha pager
flashes her number and
text I entered in the tiny field of white:
Baby hasn't moved in 24 hours.
Second call back.

Untethered

Doctor M. is driving away
from the hospital and ***will not***
come back for anyone or anything.
I continue to enter his messages
into his alpha pager,
numbers and names.
When he is done at seven,
he will erase them all and
float free as I will after my shift,
hovering over this field of tangled nettles,
fallen tree limbs covered with fungus,
upturned roots, lightning-scarred bark.

Then rising higher…we will see pools
of water, streams and meandering rivers
we never knew existed;
the narrow path I followed below,
hacking my way through underbrush,
careful where I placed each foot,
looking for pieces of open sky.

All Fall to Earth

Birds weave in and out
of each other—not quite a murmuration,
their bodies delicate and translucent.
I wish I could do the same.
If I could follow them, would I vanish
as they do into the white sky,
fading into nothingness and background
noise? I rise and fall over a strange
landscape. A spontaneous encounter,
unplanned, as most encounters
between bird and human are.
The trees' canopy brushes my face
gently. Branches reach up to grab
me but I stay afloat keeping level with birds.
As long as I don't think about it, it works.
Otherwise, I fall to earth.
Birds alight on a birch, then disperse.
I take myself home,
following a few stragglers.

First Disaster

A wall of water is moving down Main Street.
The Police Station and Town Hall are gone.
The hospital switchboard becomes
the answering service for the Red Cross
on this Saturday morning in October.
I have my first official disaster.
A couple is stranded in their home.
Where should we go? they ask.
The shelters are opening at two locations.
Evacuees need medicines and food.
Meanwhile, the hospital awakens,
patients need transports, nursing homes
want to reach the covering doctor
while the Cold River swells,
taking the houses off their foundations,
flooding fields, tearing up asphalt.

First Code

Sunday quiet pours in the front
door like honey, my limbs
feel heavy, eyelids close.
Then the code phone jangles,
red light pulsing, the receiver
becomes alive in my hands.
I handle it awkwardly,
as if it were a writhing snake.
Security STAT Adolescent Wing,
the voice commands.
I exchange code phone for the
switchboard handset and speak
into its mouthpiece
repeating these words:
Security STAT Adolescent Wing,
pronouncing STAT with a hiss,
a command like STOP! NOW! RESIST!
My voice goes everywhere—
to every unit on five floors,
to bathroom stalls, doctor's sleep room,
nurse bent over a computer,
the empty meditation room.
In the Mental Health Unit,
I imagine a young girl
scrunched in the corner
of her hospital room
yells *fuck you* at my voice.

Security

Our only guard is belligerent
after his evening in the ER.
He should be taken in a field and shot,
referring to the man he guarded all night
on a stand-by.
He tells me police are no better
than social workers.
I am thinking: better than security guards
who are not social workers
with a bent for violence.

He opens doors on weekends:
for the courier who arrives with an iron box,
for the teachers of classes:
yoga for pregnant women, siblings of infants,
teens' court, stop smoking clinic,
nurses who need supplies.

Where are you? I ask, speaking into the radio,
then I hear his heavy breathing.
He is running between floors.
Will I have to call a code on him?
I hope he answers and is not in a dead zone.

The Hospital as Halfway House

Halfway between home and nursing home,
halfway between life and death,
halfway between prison and home
or wherever one lives after prison,
the woman that a driver
from the County Jail drops off
on Saturday morning with a twenty-dollar bill.
She has no reservations at the hospital,
her belongings in a single plastic bag.
I've made mistakes, she says softly.
We let her call her son who lives out of state.
Self-possessed with a quiet dignity,
she impresses us and the nurse leader
who would later say she acted
    appropriately.
She is a well-mannered homeless woman
who once was a nurse.
The taxi will take her to the Community Kitchen.
She is not ready to be admitted to the ER,
she tells the nurse.
Her body looks like a tight ball of stress
that cannot be hugged away.

Code Red

A series of events set in motion
by a smoldering rice sock
warming in a microwave on the ICU unit.
Code Red South Building 3rd floor ICU unit.
Three times I announce the code
into the tan handset,
two times on the radio,
once into the pagers.
I cannot call it back
despite the nurse's request.
The Code Red will be executed
to its conclusion: doors close
on the floors.
Heavily suited firemen emerge
from their fire trucks.
The security guard waits at the front door.
The engineer resets the alarm,
an hour from start to finish,
after which the rice sock will be draped
over the nurse's aching neck.

Panic Buttons

Occupational health has one, the registration desk,
orthopedic office, all of which are closed nights.
But our office open 24/7
does not have a panic alarm.
A man who looks like he just rolled
out of bed is doing a walk-about
in the lobby, coming closer and closer
to my glass window.
How can I call security on the radio,
without this man seeing me?
I am panicking
in my office without a panic button.
His mouth is moving, a chant, perhaps,
prayer or a string of obscenities.
If I keep on my headset with loose-fitting
ear pieces and pretend to answer calls
he may leave, which he does,
right out of the front door, walking
into the frigid winter air with no coat on.

Tonight the security guard feels threatening.
He lingers in my office after a routine check,
standing behind me, waiting for me to turn,
for me to acknowledge his presence.
I want him to leave but he won't.
He comes closer.
I tell him he is requested for a stand-by in the ER.
Only then does he leave the office,
slamming the door behind him.

Calling Codes

Simplex™ sounds like a typewriter,
scrolls out paper with print:
red letters squeezed together
note the locations for fire
or troubles in the system.
C-CURE™ sounds like a high-pitched ambulance,
until I acknowledge and close it down.
Code Red activates flashing disco lights
and a woman's automated voice
perfectly modulated and calm
announces the code.
I want to be that voice.
She conveys seriousness without panic.
This is the art of the job
if there is any art here.

I ask my boss how to prioritize:
what if I get a Lifeline™ call and Code Red
at the same time?
What do I do first?
Code Red takes precedence over everything
she answers smugly.
She knows her protocols.

The Code Red I announce
travels to the bathroom stalls, cubicles,
x-ray changing rooms, IV suites,
gym pool area where
the *Twinges and Hinges*
senior group is doing pool aerobics,
doctor rooms where patients
lie on cold examining tables,
the woman's legs splayed,
feet into cold steel stirrups.

My voice may be the last
thing the OR patient
hears as she drifts into her Versed™ sleep.

It is: "ATTENTION PLEASE!"
and not "May I have your attention please."
It is not a choice that you listen.
I calibrate my voice to reassure the listeners:
we have the situation under control,
we are following our protocols.
Machines will continue their work.
Scopes will continue to probe, knives will cut,
the nurse will continue to inflate
the blood pressure cuff,
then it will be released.

Lifeline™ Calls

I can hear the subtle click
before the alarm sounds.
*This is the Lifeline™ operator,
are you all right, Virginia?*
My voice is loud enough
that the entire lobby can hear.
A small voice answers
back from some distant room.
It sounds as distant from the Earth
as the moon.
Her voice, young-sounding
for a 95-year old, complains,
*They are always testing me,
even in the middle of the night!*

Another voice is silent when
the signal comes in.
Has she fallen? Is she dying?
She lives on a country road
twenty-five minutes from here.
I read her medical history:
heart attack, ten medications, and
two responders I cannot reach.
Mutual Aid will send an ambulance.

When I finally look up,
a man is standing at my glass window.
How long has he been waiting?
Sunday evening and the lobby is dark:
22:40:05 Greenwich Mean Time.
I open the window smudged
with fingerprints and he blurts out:

*My wife just died and I need
to reach our children, where
can I get cell phone coverage?*

Weekend Call Sheets

Hospice on pink sheets,
urology calls on yellow,
purple for Red Cross.
Good Morning!...a dam is breaking,
there is blood in his urine,
a hospice patient is actively dying.
Conversely, can someone be actively living?
Certainly not me, tethered to this board
for seven hours,
pressed into my seat by the weight
of emergencies.

Patient...no correct that,
Lifeline™ subscriber has fallen
the hospice client is agitated and needs medication.
From the pink home health care sheet
I read the history of a woman's dying,
from midnight to five a.m.—
dysphasia at midnight,
then gurgling noises at two,
rattling noises in her chest at three.
By five, she has stopped breathing.

A daughter calls with a message
for the hospice nurse.
Her father has passed—
fifteen minutes ago.
I give her silence, a tiny space
of time so she can continue.
I want to tell her my father
is dying but I can't.
She holds back tears
but crying would be better than words.
I am so tired of words.

The Vigil

I come close to kiss your forehead
and smell roses.
Your eye opens, revolving
in its socket, without focus,
a shade of color not your own—
bluish-brown like a polished stone.
Behind this eye, trauma resides
in a home that is shutting down.
The caretaker closes off rooms
one by one
until there is one chamber
where you will spend the night.

Overheard

My chair has three levers:
seat depth, seat height, back angle.
When I push the wrong lever,
I drop precipitously to the floor.
Oh, escapes from my lips
and a voice answers—*yes?*
A call has popped on the line
and I did not know
someone was listening to me
laughing, fragments of conversations.
Once it was about sex
and the man warned me:
Don't say another word.

Crash

The motherboard crashes at station one.
Apparently, the computer loses data,
the last page erased though I have
no memory of what I was doing last.
I bring my board back with three keystrokes,
back to the beginning with a clean screen,
enter my initials and password.
I enjoy a few seconds of quiet,
remembering to take a deep breath.
My face reflected back from the glass
window looks shrunken and oddly shaped.
Other operators pick up my dropped calls.
I can hear angry voices of a
customer/client/patient
from another operator's headset.
Sorry, sorry, sorry
I mutter between calls.

How Did You Do That?

I lean on the keyboard and hit
a combination of keys by mistake,
nothing I could ever replicate.
My screen is sideways.
I have to turn my head sideways
to read it—impossible!
I have never seen anyone do that,
the other operator giggles.
Another morning I cannot read
anything, even with my glasses on.
Am I going blind?
How can I finish my shift?
Panic sets in, maybe I can go
to the after-hours clinic and
ask about this sudden loss of vision,
when the young man I am relieving
notices I have a lens missing.
It lies on my lap and I replace
it in the frame gently.
Last Sunday, I had two headsets
wrapped around my neck.
Ready for Sunday morning? he quipped.
He programs the computers, cruises
the internet on his overnight shift.
He is very cool.
I am not.

Voices

traveling through the wire,
through the headset,
vibrating string across cochlea
bones and hammer,
translated by the cortex into words.
I supply the missing parts—
decipher the callers' pauses
into commas, dashes, or ellipses
where we both take a breath,
or that question dropped onto the middle
of the sentence when I least
expect it, an afterthought,
spoken in a soft voice
so I almost can't hear it
but it is important.
The caller who asks it,
acknowledges a possibility:
the cancer has returned, the
pain under the right scapula
is not indigestion,
the headache not a migrane.
I become a reader of voices
and when I hear my own
coming back to me from speakerphone
it sounds as if it belongs
to a snotty teenager—
not my own.

Hearing Test

She notes the tortuous turns
of my ear canal.
My stomach gurgles loudly
in this acoustically sensitive cell.
Headphones sit heavy on my head
and dig into my skull.
The tester requests that I repeat
her two-syllable words.
She adds background noises,
one sounds like a foghorn.
I am on the coast of Maine
near a secluded cove.
The fog is coming in.
Then the sound of a train
traveling through a tunnel
that is my cochlea.

Harvesting

An OR tech suited in blue
holds a bag of ice.
He is harvesting organs from a donor
and needs a key to the morgue.
I guess who it is…who it was.
He died on 4:45 on a Friday afternoon,
twenty-five years younger than I am.
His skin is rolled like sheets of parchment,
corneas punched out before
the sclera turns black.
There is a small window of time
to work in the garden of the body.

After-Life

The mortician arrives and wants
the death certificate, incomplete
as it is, with no cause of death.
He assures me he will take care
of everything.
Before he has come to my window,
he has loaded the body into his vehicle
from the morgue with a key
he is not supposed to have.
He used the stretchers that squeal
and are half-broken—reserved
for the dead.

Now we are tightening our protocols.
A body was taken before the organ harvest.
Now I need to call a nurse supervisor
before he leaves with a body.

His fingerprints will remain on the glass window,
from when he tried to remove the barrier
between me and him,
between me and the sick,
between me and the dead.

STAT

…is a life interrupted,
a word set apart in a sentence.
When I speak it, I pause before and after.
The fricative *s* morphs
into a plosive *t* like gunfire,
tongue behind the teeth,
the open vowel cut off
by a second round of gunfire.

STAT is the possibility hidden
in every admission, routine surgery.
A prank on a calm April afternoon:
to careen over a waterfall in an inflatable pool.
Two college students hear the churning of water
in their ears, a woman's voice
calling a STAT,
waking them to their own nightmare.

By ten a.m I have called three codes.
Respiratory STAT punctuates the air
with exclamation.
Dr. K to the STAT lab.
OR team for STAT c-section.
The RN First Assists are off their pagers,
one is bowling, one is shopping,
a third sitting in church.
I keep dialing numbers, leaving messages.

Utero-scopy is not STAT
but it is urgent; likewise the "lap appy."
Tell them to come in asap the doctor snaps when I ask.
After the surgical team assembles,
quiet returns to the hospital

although I am not allowed to say the
word "quiet" out loud (hospital taboo).

I return to my oxbow in the river, now flat
water and follow the river
to the mouth of the ocean,
listening for the foghorn,
waiting for a break in the morning fog.

Self-Revelation

I have no opinion, relay messages
to the *locum tenens* doctor in a neutral tone.
My phone behavior, above reproach
and discreet.
Today, the levee I have built
collapses when I ask the doctor
about *failure to thrive*.
The river that is my story begins
to flood verdant pastures and oxbows
where I had thrived before,
where I recited the poetry of Coleridge
and Yeats and wrote poems.
At the switchboard, I speak another
language: driven by machines,
composed of Latinate roots, prefix and suffix.
River's rhythm interrupted by random
events: his petit mal seizure,
genetic findings, fragile bones.
Predictable—only its constant movement
and threat of floods and rain.
My voice softens as I talk to this doctor.
He tells me to talk louder,
he wants to hear more.

Loud the Silence

I am under a trance,
no phones ringing,
no alarms on the C-CURE™ screens
no alarms on the Simplex™ panel,
which need to be acknowledged
then disabled.
Strange this silence,
absence of meaningful noise.
I forget where I am.
I am outside of the hospital's
arrhythmic heartbeat.
I become lost in a book—
Emily Dickinson's snake
slithers through pasture grass
like whiplash.
I feel someone's eyes
looking down at me, a visitor
at the window, and through their eyes
I become aware again of my surroundings:
eight phones, digital and analog,
two video screens displaying
nine areas of the hospital,
two fax machines, one copier,
two cellular phones, a conference
phone, two TTY phones,
a microphone and emergency
communication system under glass
like a museum exhibit.

For Liesbet

I type a text message for a patient
in a county nursing home:
resident has glioblastoma and dysphagia;
in need of pain meds.
Before the nurse gives her name,
I know who it is—my best friend.

I reflect back to the waterfall,
near the West River.
She brought me there three years ago.
The flecks of mica had shone like diamonds.

We sat on granite slabs
comfortable with our silence,
listening to water, imagining its source.
She took pictures, assemblages of leaves
caught in an eddy of water.
The rocks chiseled by weather and water
formed a staircase we climbed.

These photographs now hang on
the wall opposite her bed.
When I visit, she strokes her gold necklace
with the jade Buddha.
From her window, the Connecticut River is visible.
From this height, it looks flat and uninteresting
but I know that is not true.

When I leave her room I cross River Road
walk beyond the grounds of the County Nursing Home,
the farm and prison
where inmates work the rich bottomland
and walk closer to the River.

After the After-Hours Clinic Closes

and the switchboard is open for calls.
An older man is coughing up his lungs,
another is *bleeding like a stuck pig*.
Her water may have broke.
It is Sunday morning and she
needs the morning after pill
like two hours ago!
His rash is moving up his body,
her child's cast fell into the toilet,
another kid has a tick,
the prescription is not at the drugstore,
and better yet, the drugstore is
out of her medicine. Backordered?
The man's penis has been hard for hours.
I hate urology calls.
Ten feet of intestine removed from another,
she can't leave the house.
The woman had her gallbladder removed
and is now vomiting bile.
Wait…I pay attention to this!
Isn't that the surgery I am having
in two weeks?
Another father says his daughter
is having suicidal ideations,
I think he means *thoughts* and connect
him to the mental health unit.
I have to dry out a man's gruff
voice, barely audible.
I am driving my son to the ER,
he is out of control.
Please have someone meet us.
Another mother pleads:
My daughter has been raped.
Please find my daughter.

I am so sorry, I say.
My words sound hollow
as if I am in an echo chamber.
I am beginning to sound programmed
like what I imagine a telephone operator
is supposed to sound like.
Thank you, thank you, thank you,
she answers when I say *I am very sorry.*
This mother is in shock
and I am losing my voice.
It is about Lea the only message
a caller wants to leave for the doctor.
Just tell the doctor that.
She will know what I mean.
A mother wants her son's belongings,
he died in the emergency room.
A young woman is having breakthrough pain
no, correct that…breakthrough bleeding.
Before I can stop her she goes on to say
she had sex the night before and
this morning.
It sounds as if she is popping gum.
If I let her ramble, does that make
me a voyeur…
am I breaking HIPPA standards?
She is sore and I am goddamn jealous,
tethered to this work station,
sitting in this chair
with the old lady smell.

Misreads (at the Switchboard)

Department of Eternal Medicine
not to be confused with Eternal
Blessings Crematorium
opens at 8:30, not 8:00.
The nunnery is open 365 days
a year, for virgins in recovery.
Breast pump rentals available.
Two floors above, adolescent
angst lights up the board.
Nurses' heads bobble on brain stems
as they reach for stale peanut brittle
on the telemetry unit.
Hemlock Branch of Twinges
and Hinges group hit the side of the pool
knocking themselves senseless.
Rejected linens will never find a home.
Washing machines churn, creating heat.
Switchboard operators sit inside their nests,
nerve-startled by crises, codes, and trauma.
Twitter of birds inside their console
breaks out in inconsolable song,
heartbeat of the hospital—
    arrhythmic.

Late Shift

The hospital has a thousand thresholds,
each door a Station of the Cross,
each patient a pilgrim traveling
their singular Way of Sorrows.
Phones rest in their cradles.
An operator tethered to her station
opens a line to hear the hum of the phone
then severs the connection.
Three a.m. and the video cameras
scan the dark corners.
Nine screens play emptiness
save for the wolverine
who stalks the hallways.
Closed doorways mean nothing to him.
He brings the Northern cold like
tiny knives working under their skin.
Staff put on their coats and hats so
they can do their work, avoiding
his shadow.

Acknowledgments

"Harvesting" appeared online in January 2010 issue of *International Psychoanalysis*

"Late Shift" and "The Vigil" appeared online in September 2009 issue of *The Houston Literary Review*

"Weekend Call Sheets" appeared online in the Fall, 2012 issue of *Smoky Quartz Quarterly*

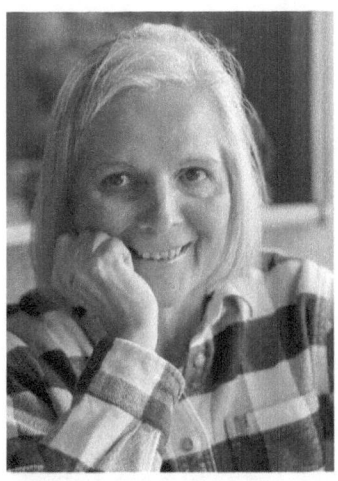

About the Author

Kathleen Fagley is a Pushcart-nominated poet whose chapbook, *How You Came to Me*, was published by *Finishing Line Press* in July 2012. Her second chapbook was published by *Concrete Wolf* in 2024. Her poems have appeared in *The Stillwater Review, Memoir Journal, Cutthroat, Nimrod Journal, Adanna: A Collection of Contemporary Love Poems,* and others. In addition, her essay on Jean Valentine's work was included with several other poets in *This World Company* published by University of Michigan in 2012, edited by Kazim Ali and John Hoppenthaler.

Her work has appeared in the following anthologies: *The Poet's Touchstone, The Best of Write Action No.2., Poets' Guide: An Anthology of New Hampshire Poets,* and the *2010 Poets' Guide to New Hampshire: More Places, More Poets.*

Having received her MFA from New England College in 2005, she became an adjunct professor at Keene State College in Poetry and Creative Non-Fiction, teaching for five years. She received the Adjunct Faculty Excellence Award in Teaching in 2019.

She was a poetry editor for the Monadnock Writers Group and an editor of the Monadnock Writers Group publication, *Shadow and Light: A Literary Anthology on Memory*, and an editor of *Amoskeag: The Journal of Southern New Hampshire University*.

She has attended the Frost Place for Advanced Poetry for four summer sessions, and the Vermont post Graduate Writer's Conference in Montpelier, Vermont, working with Leslie Ullman, Vivee Francis, Jean Beaumont, and Martha Collins, among others.

www.ingramcontent.com/pod-product-compliance
Lightning Source LLC
Chambersburg PA
CBHW030533080526
44586CB00011B/430